# How to Get The Most Out Of Your Chiropractic Care

## 289 Great Chiropractic Wellness Tips To Improve Your Life Quality

ADAM COLTON

Published by BizMove
www.bizmove.com

# Disclaimer

All the content found in this book was created for informational purposes only. The Content is not intended to be a substitute for professional medical advice, diagnosis, or treatment. Always seek the advice of your physician or other qualified health provider with any questions you may have regarding a medical condition. Never disregard professional medical advice or delay in seeking it because of something you have read in this book.

# 289 Great Chiropractic Wellness Tips To Improve Your Life Quality

Every day, people from all walks of life try to cope with issues in their back. But, these issues can become so bad that simple daily activities become too much to handle. For people in this situation, the answer is chiropractic care. If you fall in this category or just want to know more, continue reading!

1. Talk with your friends about anyone they've used for chiropractic care. Sometimes it's those close to you that know the best people to call. If you've got friends who swear by a certain doctor, then it may save you a ton of time in searching for the best one around.

2. If you are looking for a chiropractor, conduct telephone interviews with them before going to them in person. Keep in mind that potentially a majority of chiropractors engage in practices that are not scientifically backed. Talk to them on the phone to gauge their personal attitudes and patterns of practice.

3. If you are visiting a chiropractor regularly, track your progress over the first five sessions. If you aren't seeing any improvement at all after just these first few visits, you are probably wasting

your time. Look for another caregiver and then give them a try of at least three sessions.

4.  Make sure you make a wise decision when searching for a chiropractor. Just like in any profession, there are good and bad chiropractors. In fact, some chiropractors end up making your pain even worse. Therefore, it is important to carefully choose a chiropractor.

5.  Look for a chiropractor that offers a free consultation. Since you may be having regular sessions with a chiropractor, it is a good idea to know what you are getting into. Use that time to ask any questions and gauge the type of provider they are. If you feel uncomfortable at any time, you should look for someone else.

6.  Chiropractic care focuses on your skeletal and nervous system and the functioning of your brain. The central nervous system and brain control all the functions of your body, so regular chiropractic care can lead to excellent overall health. When your central nervous system is functioning properly, all of your autonomic functions, such as heartbeat, breathing and digestion work unimpeded.

7.  Research what chiropractic really is prior to going to a chiropractor. A lot of people have strange ideas about what these doctors do. They think chiropractic does strange things to your bones or muscles. It's not true. There's a lot of great information online that will help you understand the benefits of chiropractic.

8.  Always speak with a doctor before you go to get chiropractor services. You definitely want a doctor to assess your situation. This information will also be transferred to the chiropractor, which will help them better deal with your case. It could indicate that a chiropractor isn't the way to go. Your physician might see the need for different treatment.

9.  Before choosing a chiropractor, look into his or her licensing. A quality chiropractor will be licensed. If there is no official license for the doctor you are seeing, look elsewhere immediately. Remember, chiropractic is not something to fool around with. If you wonder about a person's credentials, don't take the chance.

10. To protect your spine when siting in front of a computer for long periods of time, make sure you have an ergonomic chair. A good chair

should have a backrest and adjustable arm rests which maintain good posture when seating. The chair should also let you decrease or increase height so your legs can comfortable bend at the knee while keeping your feet flat on the floor.

11. Birth processes that are used today can cause chiropractic problems in infants. Traumatic birth syndrome results when subluxation of the spine is created during birth. This causes damage to the neck and the nervous system of newborn babies. For this reason, it is very important to have your baby checked by a chiropractor early on.

12. Chiropractic care can help improve lung function in patients suffering from asthma. The nerves in your spinal cord regulate the diaphragm and the lungs. If your spine is misaligned, your lungs may not function properly. When the spine is manipulated into proper alignment, nerve supply can be restored to your lungs. Patients can see up to a 50 percent decrease in the number of asthmatic attacks by visiting a chiropractor.

13. It is easy to find good chiropractors these days. Many people use chiropractors. Chiropractic training is quite rigorous and demanding. For example, they have to know about human

anatomy and they must have 4 years of graduate training to do their jobs. Any chiropractor you go to should be trained and certified.

14. When you are standing for any length of time, place one foot slightly in the front of your other foot and keep your knees slightly bent and not rigidly locked. Taking this position will help to reduce the pressure on your spine and your lower back. Switch the position of your feet every few minutes to also help to keep strain from building up.

15. Before beginning any manipulation, it is important that your chiropractor discusses the benefits as well as risks associated with chiropractic care. Although chiropractic care has many benefits, there are still risks that must be considered. If a doctor does not discuss them with you, you are advised to contact a different chiropractor.

16. If you have a familial medical history of illnesses, a great chiropractor will refer you to a physician to ensure it is safe to perform chiropractic manipulations on you. This is especially important if you or any blood relatives have heart disease, diabetes or lung problems. If

you are concerned, talk with your chiropractor before starting any treatment plan.

17. If your back feels sore or tight, apply ice and heat to the area that hurts. If you use heat, try using moist heat, such as a moist heat pad or a warm shower, which is more beneficial. You can also wrap a heating pad with a damp towel and turn on the pad to create moist heat.

18. Don't just choose the chiropractor closest to you. It may be tempting to opt for the shortest drive, but it's better to opt for quality instead. A good doctor is worth the extra time in your car. Too often people find that with just a little extra time they could have had a much better experience.

19. Properly get out of your bed in the morning. Start your ascent with a nice stretch and then slowly rise out of the bed. As you begin to move, swing your legs down, supporting your body with your arms. Getting of of bed like this will prevent spinal problems.

20. If you are visiting a chiropractor regularly, track your progress over the first five sessions. If you aren't seeing any improvement at all after just these first few visits, you are probably wasting

your time. Look for another caregiver and then give them a try of at least three sessions.

21. Do you suffer from fatigue? Many times fatigue is caused by tense neck and back muscles. By repositioning your back, the nerve flow is increased which allows the muscles in your back and neck to relax allowing you to rest comfortably while you are sleeping; thus, improving your fatigue by getting the necessary rest.

22. Many types of health issues can be helped by chiropractic care. Since most nerves and muscles of the body originate in the spine, misalignment of the spine can result in various pains and health issues throughout the body. Chiropractic adjustments can be very helpful in any pain related to nerves or muscles.

23. Make sure your back is supported when writing on a flat surface. Try supporting your head with one of your hands. You need to take breaks often when writing. You should get up and stretch your body during these breaks. Lastly, make sure the chair you're sitting in is comfortable.

24. Don't get frustrated if the pain returns after a few days. You'll usually get a chiropractic surge of energy following an adjustment. Your body will feel great! But that may wear off after a few days. This is why multiple treatments are often needed to get your body back in the shape it needs to be. Over time, your body will feel better and better.

25. Don't be surprised if after a chiropractic adjustment that your body feels worse. It will go away. For some people, treatment gives them an immediate boost of energy, but for others it can seem to worsen the issue. Really give it time. The pain will subside, and you'll start feeling a lot better.

26. Chiropractic care is not just for people that have back and neck issues. It can help your immune system as well. Your nervous system can be affected by bones in your spinal column that are misaligned. Because the nervous system is in control of cell, organ and tissue function, if it gets impacted it can make your health go wrong. If you correct the core issue, the other issues will correct themselves.

27. If your chiropractor wants to put you through neck manipulation, ask him for a clear

justification. Because neck manipulation puts you at risk of damage to the vertebral artery, it should be a last resort and should only take place when there is a pressing need, so if your chiropractor uses this for all patients, go to another one instead.

28. Many people are afraid of visiting a chiropractor; however, chiropractic care can help a plethora of ailments, including back pain, asthma, digestive issues and high blood pressure. A chiropractor can help you not only feel better, but can also keep you from contracting bacterial infections. This is because chiropractic care has been shown to boost the body's natural immunity.

29. When you are feeling back discomfort at home, think about applying ice to the affected area. Put cubes of ice into a plastic bag or apply an ice pack to your back. You can also by ice packs in a gel form that you can freeze and re-use multiple times.

30. When you have back pain and are undergoing chiropractic treatment, make sure you stretch your back before you get out of bed in the morning. Raise slowly to a seated position, and support your weight with your arms while

swinging your legs around to the floor. This can keep your spine from developing further injury.

31. To avoid back pain after a night's sleep, make sure that you do not sleep on your stomach. Sleep on the side, with a pillow in between the knees and another beneath your neck and head, or sleep on your back, with pillows under your shoulders and head as well as your knees.

32. Your chiropractor should not be attempting any spinal manipulations before ordering a diagnostic x-ray or MRI so the nature of your ailment is very clear. A full exam and X-rays can help you get proper chiropractic care. Don't even consider allowing any treatment before your chiropractor has studied all your x-rays and any other appropriate tests. Instead, find another chiropractor.

33. When you experience back pain at home, you can use ice or heat to deal with the discomfort. Both methods have advantages and drawbacks, though. Ice brings swelling down but can make your muscles tighter. Heat relaxes those muscles but can cause swelling. Alternate between the two methods for the best results.

34. Talk with your friends about anyone they've used for chiropractic care. Sometimes it's those close to you that know the best people to call. If you've got friends who swear by a certain doctor, then it may save you a ton of time in searching for the best one around.

35. Did you know that chiropractic care can boost your body's immunity? If your spine is compromised, it may screw with your immune system. If your spine is correctly aligned, the nervous system will get more blood. This blood flow increases your body's ability to fight off infection.

36. Don't just choose the chiropractor closest to you. It may be tempting to opt for the shortest drive, but it's better to opt for quality instead. A good doctor is worth the extra time in your car. Too often people find that with just a little extra time they could have had a much better experience.

37. When you are lifting items from the floor, you should never bend down with your back and pick them up. Doing this can cause damage to your back, so avoid it at all costs. The best method for picking up things is to bend your knees, squat and lift it up.

38. If you are visiting a chiropractor regularly, track your progress over the first five sessions. If you aren't seeing any improvement at all after just these first few visits, you are probably wasting your time. Look for another caregiver and then give them a try of at least three sessions.

39. When looking for a new chiropractor, see if you can set up a consultation with them. Many of them are more than willing to meet with you via a free consultation. Try getting as much as you can from this visit. This can help see whether or not they are right for your needs.

40. Before you consult a chiropractor, make sure a competent medical practitioner diagnoses your problem. Do not rely on the diagnosis of a chiropractor. Even though there are chiropractors who are know enough to give a proper diagnosis, it is hard for a consumer to determine who that can be. As additional precaution, ask your chiropractor to talk about your care with your doctor.

41. Stay away from chiropractors who market about the warning signs indicating the necessity for chiropractic treatment, who claim to be able to cure diseases, who want you to sign a long-term

contract for treatment, market a regular course of preventive treatments, or use fear tactics. Those are just after your money.

42. When looking for a chiropractor, ask those you are considering about the conditions they treat. Chiropractors that are treating things other than back discomforts or other musculoskeletal problems are going outside of what will be seen as effective. You can more readily trust chiropractors that stick within these lines.

43. Did you know you can receive chiropractic care while your pregnant? Many women do not realize how beneficial this can be. The added pregnancy weight can put pressure on your back and neck causing discomfort. Studies have shown that manipulations by a chiropractor can relieve up to 85 percent of back pain associated with pregnancy.

44. If your back causes your problems, avoid sleeping on your stomach. This will pull your spine away from its natural alignment. It is better to lie with pillows supporting your shoulders and knees while you sleep. A rolled up towel can be added under the neck. This will protect the natural curve in your spine.

45. Many people with back issues sleep on their sides. To do this without experiencing further pain, keep your neck on the same level with the remainder of the spine, and keep a pillow beneath your head and neck. Also place a cushion between the knees, and bend them to reduce lower back strain.

46. To avoid back pain after a night's sleep, make sure that you do not sleep on your stomach. Sleep on the side, with a pillow in between the knees and another beneath your neck and head, or sleep on your back, with pillows under your shoulders and head as well as your knees.

47. When you are applying heat to your back, moist heat is best. You can hop into a warm shower and stand beneath the hot water, or you can put a heating pad in a plastic sack. Cover the sack with a damp cloth, and then turn on the heating pad to generate moist heat.

48. If you are experiencing severe back pain and regularly do crunches or sit-ups to build core strength, it's time to find other core exercises, because those two can worsen the pain. Yoga's plank position is a great alternative, and is easy to master if you find online videos demonstrating it.

49. To maintain a healthy neck and back, make sure that you don't sleep on your stomach anymore. This position forces you to turn your head in one direction or the other, leading to neck strain. Better choices include sleeping on your back, with a cushion beneath your knees, or on the side with a cushion between the knees.

50. Never take a child to a chiropractor who does not normally treat children. Children are still growing and their skeletons and musculature are quite different from adults. If you think your child needs chiropractic care, seek out a chiropractor who normally treats children and ask them for their professional opinion.

51. To maintain a healthy spine while you are asleep, you have to maintain the natural curves of its structure. You can sleep on one side, with a cushion between the knees, or on your back, putting a cushion beneath your knees. In either position, also put a small cushion beneath your head, and position it so it also supports the neck.

52. Ask your doctor what type of stretching he or she recommends between visits. Half of chiropractic care happens on the outside of the office. It's up to you, in your own home, to make the best of your time with the chiropractor. Be

sure to stretch and exercise. It'll make a big difference.

53. Don't get frustrated if the pain returns after a few days. You'll usually get a chiropractic surge of energy following an adjustment. Your body will feel great! But that may wear off after a few days. This is why multiple treatments are often needed to get your body back in the shape it needs to be. Over time, your body will feel better and better.

54. Do you have high blood pressure? Recent studies have proven that manipulating a specific vertebrae in the neck can be just as effective as taking two different blood pressure medications. Manipulation of the vertebra decreases nerve pressure that regulates blood pressure.

55. Be wary of any chiropractic clinic that tries to get you to purchase a package of treatments. A qualified professional will not need to sell packages of treatments to get your business. If you feel you can make full use of all the treatments, check out the clinic carefully before signing a contract.

56. Don't expect a miracle cure. While chiropractic can do a lot, one treatment isn't going to all of a

sudden make you pain free. Just like any treatment regimen, it's going to take time, dedication, and patience. Expect to have multiple trips to the chiropractor before you start seeing lasting results.

57. Research what chiropractic really is prior to going to a chiropractor. A lot of people have strange ideas about what these doctors do. They think chiropractic does strange things to your bones or muscles. It's not true. There's a lot of great information online that will help you understand the benefits of chiropractic.

58. Avoid chiropractors that try to load you up with dietary pills, herbal and homeopathic products. They are likely just trying to upsell you based on products they offer and cannot be trusted. You can get this advice from a nutritionist or a doctor.

59. If your chiropractor offers you herbal supplements as part of the overall care, it may be a sign that your doctor is not on the up and up. Herbal supplements are not something you'd typically see being offered by licensed chiropractors. Do your homework here and look to another chiropractor if you have concerns.

60. If your chiropractor wants to put you through neck manipulation, ask him for a clear justification. Because neck manipulation puts you at risk of damage to the vertebral artery, it should be a last resort and should only take place when there is a pressing need, so if your chiropractor uses this for all patients, go to another one instead.

61. Many people are afraid of visiting a chiropractor; however, chiropractic care can help a plethora of ailments, including back pain, asthma, digestive issues and high blood pressure. A chiropractor can help you not only feel better, but can also keep you from contracting bacterial infections. This is because chiropractic care has been shown to boost the body's natural immunity.

62. A newborn chiropractic check is an excellent idea to be certain your baby is not suffering from Traumatic Birth Syndrome (TBS). Injuries to the spine and brain stem that occur during the birth process have been known to cause many neurological problems. TBS may also lead to sudden infant death syndrome.

63. Be careful when a chiropractor, he should be careful with your neck. There are two arteries n the neck vertebrae that are threaded throughout

it, and that can make them kink. This would normally be okay; however, if it is stretched and turned suddenly, the artery linings can be torn. The end result can be a clot that produces a stroke.

64. Before beginning treatment, a chiropractor will check for injuries using either an MRI or x-rays. A comprehensive evaluation, with diagnostic images, helps to ensure you are getting quality care. If the chiropractor doesn't perform these tests, do not allow him to manipulate your spine. Instead, make an appointment with another chiropractor.

65. When you experience back pain at home, you can use ice or heat to deal with the discomfort. Both methods have advantages and drawbacks, though. Ice brings swelling down but can make your muscles tighter. Heat relaxes those muscles but can cause swelling. Alternate between the two methods for the best results.

66. To strengthen your core without damaging your back, take sit-ups and crunches out of the equation, because those movements can worsen the pain you feel in your back. Try the plank pose from yoga instead. This involves lying down on your stomach and then raising the body

so that you balance on toes and hands, as in the top of a push-up. Hold this plank as long as you can.

67. When you sit down, you need to have your knees up higher than the hips. Do not over straighten your back or slouch. Your back should curve naturally. If you are in a chair that has wheels, you can spin around to change your position to help take away strain on your back.

68. Before making an appointment with chiropractor, contact your insurance company and find out whether or not chiropractic care is covered under your plan. By understanding which costs are covered and which are not, you can avoid any unwelcome surprises when it comes time to pay for the services you have received.

69. Don't expect miracles after one visit to the chiropractors. You might feel relieved after seeing a chiropractor, but you can only really heal your problem if you continue to see a chiropractor. Be sure to follow your chiropractors recommendations and keep your appointments. If you don't follow the regimen, you may not like the results of your treatment.

70. Some people with chiropractic issues think they should avoid all exercises. Not only is this false, but some exercising is actually good for the back; it helps strengthens muscles in the back. So, if you have chiropractic issues and would like to exercise, a good solution is to wear a back brace and listen to your body when it says it has had enough.

71. If you're trying to find a good chiropractor, you may want to speak with a primary care doctor to figure out who a good provider is. Even if referrals aren't required, a physician might recommend a better person for your needs.

72. Chiropractic care supports nature in helping you attain vibrant health. Your body is capable of self healing when your skeletal structure is properly aligned and your central nervous system is in tip top condition. Your chiropractor knows how to make proper adjustments to stimulate excellent overall healing and health.

73. To find a reputable chiropractor, look for one who limits his practice to the conservative handling of back discomfort as well as other musculoskeletal issues. Ask your general practitioner for a referral to one that fits this criterion and has a reputation for being

trustworthy. This will weed out a lot of the quacks.

74. Steer clear of any chiropractor who claims that chiropractic can cure certain diseases. There's no proof whatsoever that chiropractic can do any such thing. Any person saying so is essentially a quack just after your money. Do yourself a favor and look elsewhere for the quality care that you deserve.

75. Make sure that you don't sign any contracts with a chiropractor who orders or performs X-ray exams as a routine strategy with all patients. The majority of patients who visit a chiropractor have no need of X-rays. Full-spine X-rays are particularly hazardous, as they mean significant radiation exposure and have little diagnostic worth.

76. Did you know you can receive chiropractic care while your pregnant? Many women do not realize how beneficial this can be. The added pregnancy weight can put pressure on your back and neck causing discomfort. Studies have shown that manipulations by a chiropractor can relieve up to 85 percent of back pain associated with pregnancy.

77. When choosing a chiropractor, it is important to find one who treats the entire body. A great chiropractor will not only manipulate the spine, but will also emphasize the importance of a well-balanced diet, proper posture and exercise. All of these areas are important to your overall health and well-being.

78. Many people with back issues sleep on their sides. To do this without experiencing further pain, keep your neck on the same level with the remainder of the spine, and keep a pillow beneath your head and neck. Also place a cushion between the knees, and bend them to reduce lower back strain.

79. Before getting any spinal manipulation, a chiropractor needs to perform an MRI or full-body X-ray to rule out torn arteries, injuries, or fractured bones. This will make sure you get the necessary care. If this is not done when you visit a chiropractor for the first time, you shouldn't allow him or her to do anything. You probably should seek the services of another chiropractor.

80. Be wary of chiropractors who suggest long-term care without any goals. You shouldn't have to be dependent on a chiropractor for the rest of your life. Don't waste your time and money. If a

chiropractor suggests long-term care, they should have some sort of a goal in mind for your body.

81. Pregnancy can be one of the most anticipated events of a woman's life. Unfortunately it is often accompanied by pain and discomfort caused by the strain pregnancy places on the joints of your body. Regular chiropractic care and reduce back pain and result in shorter labor times. Visit your chiropractor for a more comfortable pregnancy.

82. When you are applying heat to your back, moist heat is best. You can hop into a warm shower and stand beneath the hot water, or you can put a heating pad in a plastic sack. Cover the sack with a damp cloth, and then turn on the heating pad to generate moist heat.

83. Ask a chiropractor about alternate treatments if chiropractic care does not seem to be helping. Some pain can be ongoing and downright debilitating. If seeing a chiropractor has not gotten rid of the worst of your pain, ask about alternatives. Medication or even surgery could be necessary. Explore your options.

84. To strengthen your core without damaging your back, take sit-ups and crunches out of the

equation, because those movements can worsen the pain you feel in your back. Try the plank pose from yoga instead. This involves lying down on your stomach and then raising the body so that you balance on toes and hands, as in the top of a push-up. Hold this plank as long as you can.

85. One of the great benefits of chiropractic care is that it promotes proper nerve supply, thereby helping to boost your immune system. A misaligned spinal cord messes with your nervous system, and this "subluxation" is not good for your immune system. Thanks to chiropractic care fixing this, your nerves, organs and cells can function correctly.

86. Make sure you protect your back when sleeping. If you like sleeping on your side, keep your neck leveled with your spine by placing a pillow under your neck and head. You can relieve the strain on the lower back by placing a pillow between your knees and bending them. To prevent your body from rolling forward, have a pillow close to your chest.

87. Chiropractic care is one of the most effective methods of treating subluxation. When a vertebra is subluxated, the discs and vertebra

shift and tip from one side to another. This causes the entire spine to bend and curve. Early chiropractic treatment can be very helpful in correcting this condition and avoiding surgery.

88. Make sure your back is supported when writing on a flat surface. Try supporting your head with one of your hands. You need to take breaks often when writing. You should get up and stretch your body during these breaks. Lastly, make sure the chair you're sitting in is comfortable.

89. Chiropractic care focuses on your skeletal and nervous system and the functioning of your brain. The central nervous system and brain control all the functions of your body, so regular chiropractic care can lead to excellent overall health. When your central nervous system is functioning properly, all of your autonomic functions, such as heartbeat, breathing and digestion work unimpeded.

90. Do you have high blood pressure? Studies show that vertebrae manipulation is more effective than blood pressure medications. The manipulation lets the blood supply flow freely.

91. When you are researching potential chiropractors, be sure to ask what types of conditions they treat. Chiropractors go beyond limits of their effectiveness at times when treating something other than musculoskeletal issues and back pain. Practitioners who stick with the basics tend to be more effective.

92. If you're dealing with back pain issues, sleeping on your stomach isn't a good idea. It results in your spine being pushed out of proper position. Roll over on your back, instead, and support your shoulders and knees with pillows. Additionally, roll a towel up and place it under your neck. These techniques keep your spine's curves protected.

93. Get up slowly in the morning, especially if you are dealing with back pain. Stretch your arms and legs, rise to a sitting position slowly and lower your feet gently to the floor.

94. Be wary of chiropractors who suggest long-term care without any goals. You shouldn't have to be dependent on a chiropractor for the rest of your life. Don't waste your time and money. If a chiropractor suggests long-term care, they should have some sort of a goal in mind for your body.

95. To strengthen your core without damaging your back, take sit-ups and crunches out of the equation, because those movements can worsen the pain you feel in your back. Try the plank pose from yoga instead. This involves lying down on your stomach and then raising the body so that you balance on toes and hands, as in the top of a push-up. Hold this plank as long as you can.

96. You may think office workers couldn't experience as much pain as laborers, but they can actually experience more. Tight hamstrings are a huge cause of pain in the lower back. By standing up, the hamstring muscle pulls on the pelvis, which can cause pain in the spine. Stretching your hamstrings daily helps to combat this.

97. To help your neck relax from a day at the office, use the headrest in your car. The natural direction for the neck to point while you are using your computer is down, so counteract that by pointing your chin up and leaning your head back while driving. This gives your neck muscles a break from the long day.

98. After visiting a chiropractor it is important to eat a diet filled with vegetables. This is because of the vitamins and minerals found in vegetables.

To get the most from your vegetables, eat them raw. Eating a diet rich in vegetables also helps you lose excess body weight which can contribute to back pain.

99. Use your rear view mirror as a guide to good posture in the car. Sit in your vehicle and put your seat up in a good posture position that keeps your back straight. Adjust your mirror for this viewing angle. Once this is done, don't move it. Each time you drive, adjust your posture to use the mirror properly.

100.  If you want to keep spine and neck pain to a minimum, make sure that you get significant amounts of activity each day. The more time you spend in one consistent position, the more likely you are to experience back pain. Activity leads to more flexible muscles, reducing your musculoskeletal problems.

101.  Try to buy shoes that assist with managing back pain. Some people don't wear the right shoes for certain activities. For example, if you have the wrong shoes for running, you can injure yourself. The same applies to work situations. Shoes that are are comfortable and which support good posture are important. Find shoe stores that can help you get proper shoes.

102.    If you can afford it, visit a chiropractor who will x-ray you before beginning treatment. Many chiropractors accept walk-ins and offer to simply "adjust you". This is far from the most beneficial treatment you could be receiving. A first appointment should involve a thorough examination and a discussion of some sort of treatment plan.

103.    When you are lifting items from the floor, you should never bend down with your back and pick them up. Doing this can cause damage to your back, so avoid it at all costs. The best method for picking up things is to bend your knees, squat and lift it up.

104.    Asking your physician about recommended chiropractors is a good way to start. They will likely know a good one.

105.    Don't go to one chiropractic appointment with the idea of skipping all the others. Chiropractic is something that you need to follow through on. Most issues take many sessions to work through. You need to be prepared to give of your time. This also means creating a budget for these sessions.

106.   Focus on good posture while sitting. Arms and legs should be bent at a 90 degree angle and feet should be lined up directly under the knees. Slouching or putting your feet under your chair can cause stress on hamstring and your lower back. Sit up straight and keep your back in line.

107.   If your chiropractor offers you herbal supplements as part of the overall care, it may be a sign that your doctor is not on the up and up. Herbal supplements are not something you'd typically see being offered by licensed chiropractors. Do your homework here and look to another chiropractor if you have concerns.

108.   To protect your spine when siting in front of a computer for long periods of time, make sure you have an ergonomic chair. A good chair should have a backrest and adjustable arm rests which maintain good posture when seating. The chair should also let you decrease or increase height so your legs can comfortable bend at the knee while keeping your feet flat on the floor.

109.   When it is time to research chiropractors, make sure to inquire about their specialties. A chiropractor is overstepping his bounds if he tries to treat conditions other than

musculoskeletal issues. The people that just stick to the main areas are those who you can trust.

110.    When looking for a new chiropractor, ask your friends and family for advice. You can generally expect an honest answer from friends and family. Ask them who they see and how much they pay for a visit. It's often wise to visit a professional that someone you trust has had personal experience with.

111.    Many people are afraid of visiting a chiropractor; however, chiropractic care can help a plethora of ailments, including back pain, asthma, digestive issues and high blood pressure. A chiropractor can help you not only feel better, but can also keep you from contracting bacterial infections. This is because chiropractic care has been shown to boost the body's natural immunity.

112.    A newborn chiropractic check is an excellent idea to be certain your baby is not suffering from Traumatic Birth Syndrome (TBS). Injuries to the spine and brain stem that occur during the birth process have been known to cause many neurological problems. TBS may also lead to sudden infant death syndrome.

113.    Find something to stand on if you need to reach for something that is up high and difficult to get to. Standing on tip toe and straining to get an object at above shoulder height puts a real strain on your body. It can lead to problems with your back as well as your shoulders.

114.    A competent chiropractor needs to study a complete x-ray work-up before treatment begins. It is important to discover any conditions which could be worsened by spinal manipulation. Once you've been properly examined, you'll be able to get the kind of care you need. If you see a chiropractor who skips this step, say no to any manipulations. Instead, make an appointment with another chiropractor.

115.    It is hard to stand up for long periods of time without harming your back. If you need to do this, place a foot on a stool or low shelf to reduce lower back strain. If that isn't possible, shift the body and move as much as possible.

116.    Lifting heavy objects is one of the most common sources of chiropractic pain. Whether you're lifting a bag of dog food, your toddler, or a pile of laundry, bend at your knees (instead of your back), and make sure that you hold that

load near your stomach. Lift with the core and legs, rather than your back.

117.   Don't sit or stand with your back hunched over for prolonged periods of time. This position actually places even more stress on the back and spine, which are already under extreme pressure as it is. If you need to be hunched over, have a few breaks and make sure to change your position when you can.

118.   To strengthen your core without damaging your back, take sit-ups and crunches out of the equation, because those movements can worsen the pain you feel in your back. Try the plank pose from yoga instead. This involves lying down on your stomach and then raising the body so that you balance on toes and hands, as in the top of a push-up. Hold this plank as long as you can.

119.   When dealing with items that are too heavy or large for you to lift, consider pushing them. You can lean your body against the item and push but be sure that it cannot not fall over. You can also sit on the floor and push it with your legs.

120.　Traditional planks and side planks are great abdominal exercises for people suffering from back problems. Traditional planks require you to balance on your elbows and toes, holding your body in a flat position as long as you can. Rotate to one side, balancing on that leg and arm and holding the other arm aloft, before turning over to the other side.

121.　Many medical doctors work with alternative healers these days. Therefore, it is important to ensure that your insurance provider offers coverage for alternative therapists like a chiropractor or acupuncturist. This can make your physician's care even more effective.

122.　Talk with your friends about anyone they've used for chiropractic care. Sometimes it's those close to you that know the best people to call. If you've got friends who swear by a certain doctor, then it may save you a ton of time in searching for the best one around.

123.　If you decide to use a chiropractor, check their references before you even make an appointment. There are lots of sincere chiropractors, but there are some who try to sell you all kinds of non-chiropractic merchandise. Check on the internet for reviews and obtain references from other medical professionals if possible.

124.	The way you sleep can affect your back. One good idea would be to get a towel rolled up so you can place it under the neck when it's bed time. These items allow your head to tilt downwards, while a regular pillow lifts the head upwards.

125.	Before you consult a chiropractor, make sure a competent medical practitioner diagnoses your problem. Do not rely on the diagnosis of a chiropractor. Even though there are chiropractors who are know enough to give a proper diagnosis, it is hard for a consumer to determine who that can be. As additional precaution, ask your chiropractor to talk about your care with your doctor.

126.	To find a reputable chiropractor, look for one who limits his practice to the conservative handling of back discomfort as well as other musculoskeletal issues. Ask your general practitioner for a referral to one that fits this criterion and has a reputation for being trustworthy. This will weed out a lot of the quacks.

127.    Don't go to one chiropractic appointment with the idea of skipping all the others. Chiropractic is something that you need to follow through on. Most issues take many sessions to work through. You need to be prepared to give of your time. This also means creating a budget for these sessions.

128.    To find a reputable chiropractor, ask about treatment methods. Chiropractors who use scientifically based methods use ice packs or heat as well as ultrasound treatments and similar strategies to those used by physical therapists. Along with an exercise program at home, this treatment should yield significant advancement within just a handful of visits.

129.    Keep your feet stabilized to help your spine. Wear proper shoes. If you have foot and back problems, try asking about a foot scan. Once they find the issue, you can get a recommendation to a shoe store that specializes in proper footwear. You may also want to look at spinal pelvic stabilizers. These are made to fit your specific foot imbalance. Wearing the right pair of shoes can make a world of difference with your back health.

130. Ask your personal doctor for recommendations on the best chiropractor for your issue. Your doctor may know multiple chiropractors, and there may be the perfect one for your condition available. This can save you a lot of time in searching, and it may even get you an appointment quicker than if you cold-called.

131. Did you know you can receive chiropractic care while your pregnant? Many women do not realize how beneficial this can be. The added pregnancy weight can put pressure on your back and neck causing discomfort. Studies have shown that manipulations by a chiropractor can relieve up to 85 percent of back pain associated with pregnancy.

132. Beware of chiropractors who claim to fix all your problems with just one adjustment. This type of chiropractor will try to convince you that you do not need your OBGYN, doctor or psychologist because he can do everything for you. A good doctor will know their limit and will not mind working as part of an integrated group of doctors.

133. Using heat for back pain may do more harm than good. Heat can worsen joint, muscle, and ligament inflammation in the area. Try using ice

instead. A regular cold pack, ice in a damp towel, or frozen vegetable bags work well. You should generally do this for the first three days of minor back pain. Keep the treatments between 10 and 15 minutes each. Make sure you keep a damp cloth or towel between the ice and the painful area.

134.    When you experience back pain at home, you can use ice or heat to deal with the discomfort. Both methods have advantages and drawbacks, though. Ice brings swelling down but can make your muscles tighter. Heat relaxes those muscles but can cause swelling. Alternate between the two methods for the best results.

135.    Your chiropractor should explain the treatment plan he will be performing before beginning any manipulation. Also, he should go over the expected outcome of such treatment as well as how long you should find relief after each manipulation. Finally, the doctor should discuss the overall cost of treatment and the number of treatments you need.

136.    Never take a child to a chiropractor who does not normally treat children. Children are still growing and their skeletons and musculature are quite different from adults. If you think your

child needs chiropractic care, seek out a chiropractor who normally treats children and ask them for their professional opinion.

137.    If you have to spend a lot of time sitting at work, make sure that you do not cross your legs. Keep both feet parallel to one another and situated on the floor. If your legs are too short for this to work, prop them on a foot rest or a box to reduce lower back strain.

138.    When trying to find a chiropractor, make sure that you ensure that your insurance company approves chiropractic care. Many insurance companies require a physician referral before they will cover chiropractic care. Additionally, many insurance companies limit the number of visits to a chiropractor each year. Therefore, it is important that you talk with your insurance company.

139.    If you have problems with your back, it is never a good idea to sleep while lying on your stomach. Even if this is a comfortable position for you, it can result in damage to the vertebrae. This is because there is no spinal support when lying in that position.

140.    Call your insurance company before going to your chiropractor. No every insurance plan covers chiropractic care. Make sure you know what your insurance covers prior to being surprised afterwards. Be sure to also ask how many appointments you are allowed to have in any given year. There are often maximums.

141.    Make sure your back is supported when writing on a flat surface. Try supporting your head with one of your hands. You need to take breaks often when writing. You should get up and stretch your body during these breaks. Lastly, make sure the chair you're sitting in is comfortable.

142.    When looking for a chiropractor, try asking a friend or family member for a recommendation. You should try focusing on asking the people that share similar needs and views on health with you. Try finding out what you can from them. Ask them about the chiropractor, their fees, staff, office, offered services, schedule, etc.

143.    Tell your chiropractor about any pain you are having, even if the pain may not seem related to an aching back. The nerves in your back can cause pains in lots of unexpected areas. You may get shooting pains in the soles of your feet.

There may be tingling prickles on your legs. All of these can be related to a back issue, and your chiropractor needs to know about them.

144.    Focus on good posture while sitting. Arms and legs should be bent at a 90 degree angle and feet should be lined up directly under the knees. Slouching or putting your feet under your chair can cause stress on hamstring and your lower back. Sit up straight and keep your back in line.

145.    Remember that chiropractors should not also hawk a bunch of new age remedies. Chiropractors who endorse such products are likely charlatans. Nutritionist and medical doctors are the best professionals for this type of advice.

146.    Chiropractors believe that giving birth while lying on your back can cause spinal damage to your newborn baby. Additionally, if the doctor pulls the baby from the birth canal the spine could be damaged. For this reason, chiropractors recommend giving birth in an upright position and allowing the delivery to progress naturally.

147.    When you are feeling back discomfort at home, think about applying ice to the affected area. Put cubes of ice into a plastic bag or apply

an ice pack to your back. You can also by ice packs in a gel form that you can freeze and re-use multiple times.

148.    Sleeping on your back is the best way to keep your back from feeling pain. To complement chiropractic care, put a pillow beneath the shoulders and head, and roll up a towel to place beneath your neck, and then place a pillow beneath your knees. This keeps your three primary curves supported.

149.    To avoid back pain after a night's sleep, make sure that you do not sleep on your stomach. Sleep on the side, with a pillow in between the knees and another beneath your neck and head, or sleep on your back, with pillows under your shoulders and head as well as your knees.

150.    Pregnancy can be one of the most anticipated events of a woman's life. Unfortunately it is often accompanied by pain and discomfort caused by the strain pregnancy places on the joints of your body. Regular chiropractic care and reduce back pain and result in shorter labor times. Visit your chiropractor for a more comfortable pregnancy.

151.    When lifting things, never twist as you are lifting. Twisting while you are lifting is dangerous because your muscles are straining and your spine is under pressure. This puts you at risk for sudden back spasm or pulled ligaments and tendons which can severe pain that can last for days.

152.    Your chiropractor should explain the treatment plan he will be performing before beginning any manipulation. Also, he should go over the expected outcome of such treatment as well as how long you should find relief after each manipulation. Finally, the doctor should discuss the overall cost of treatment and the number of treatments you need.

153.    To strengthen your core without damaging your back, take sit-ups and crunches out of the equation, because those movements can worsen the pain you feel in your back. Try the plank pose from yoga instead. This involves lying down on your stomach and then raising the body so that you balance on toes and hands, as in the top of a push-up. Hold this plank as long as you can.

154.    Ask your chiropractor about the different techniques they use. Chiropractors are often

versed in several techniques for alleviating pain. Do some research for yourself and discuss your options with your chiropractor. Ask them for their opinion on what would be best for you and weigh that opinion against your own.

155.    Acid reflux, gas and heartburn can be caused by a misaligned spine. The nerves running through the thoracic area of the spine control the stomach functions and can cause these and other digestive disorders. When a chiropractor adjusts your spine, the nerve flow to the stomach is aligned which helps improve your digestion.

156.    If you feel tense prior to getting chiropractic care, ask your doctor for some heating pads or warm towels. These should be placed on your back for five to ten minutes prior to treatment. This will loosen up your back, making it much more amenable to the stretching the doctor will put it through.

157.    Some people with chiropractic issues think they should avoid all exercises. Not only is this false, but some exercising is actually good for the back; it helps strengthens muscles in the back. So, if you have chiropractic issues and would like to exercise, a good solution is to wear a back

brace and listen to your body when it says it has had enough.

158.    Being pregnant can lead to subluxation of the spine for a number of reasons. The sudden gain in weight and change of posture can cause problems and spinal pain. Additionally, when you are pregnant, your sleep habits and positions may change. On top of all that, your ligaments will naturally loosen to accommodate your growing baby. All this adds ups to some very good reasons for chiropractic care during pregnancy.

159.    Receiving chiropractic care during pregnancy makes for an easier pregnancy and quicker recovery. Good chiropractic care can help you avoid damage to your own spine. It can also help your baby's central nervous system develop and function properly. Recent studies indicate that regular chiropractic care leads to a quicker and easier labor.

160.    Learn about your back problems from your chiropractor. Generally, what is happening to your spine isn't something that occurred overnight.It's usually caused by damage that has built up over time. One visit will not instantly rectify your issues. Make sure your care is

consistent with your care. This also means sticking with your treatment plan. After that plan concludes, go in for regular monthly visits to prevent recurrences or other issues.

161.   To find a reputable chiropractor, look for one who limits his practice to the conservative handling of back discomfort as well as other musculoskeletal issues. Ask your general practitioner for a referral to one that fits this criterion and has a reputation for being trustworthy. This will weed out a lot of the quacks.

162.   Don't go to one chiropractic appointment with the idea of skipping all the others. Chiropractic is something that you need to follow through on. Most issues take many sessions to work through. You need to be prepared to give of your time. This also means creating a budget for these sessions.

163.   Chiropractic care can help improve lung function in patients suffering from asthma. The nerves in your spinal cord regulate the diaphragm and the lungs. If your spine is misaligned, your lungs may not function properly. When the spine is manipulated into proper alignment, nerve supply can be restored to your lungs. Patients

can see up to a 50 percent decrease in the number of asthmatic attacks by visiting a chiropractor.

164.    To help you minimize discomfort between visits to your chiropractor, apply ice or heat to the painful area. Soreness and tightness are likely to dissipate if you apply a moist heat, through a warm shower or a damp heating pad. To give moisture to a heating pad that is dry, put it in a plastic bag and cover it with a small moist towel.

165.    Talk to your doctor about your chiropractic visits. It can be easy to see a doctor and a chiropractor, but be sure to notify your doctor about your activities. Seeing a chiropractor is healthy for you, but your doctor may wish to monitor your progress in order to adjust medication levels and to change his own treatment accordingly.

166.    When choosing a chiropractor, it is important to find one who treats the entire body. A great chiropractor will not only manipulate the spine, but will also emphasize the importance of a well-balanced diet, proper posture and exercise. All of these areas are important to your overall health and well-being.

167.    Using heat for back pain may do more harm than good. Heat can worsen joint, muscle, and ligament inflammation in the area. Try using ice instead. A regular cold pack, ice in a damp towel, or frozen vegetable bags work well. You should generally do this for the first three days of minor back pain. Keep the treatments between 10 and 15 minutes each. Make sure you keep a damp cloth or towel between the ice and the painful area.

168.    Before beginning any manipulation, it is important that your chiropractor discusses the benefits as well as risks associated with chiropractic care. Although chiropractic care has many benefits, there are still risks that must be considered. If a doctor does not discuss them with you, you are advised to contact a different chiropractor.

169.    When you experience back pain at home, you can use ice or heat to deal with the discomfort. Both methods have advantages and drawbacks, though. Ice brings swelling down but can make your muscles tighter. Heat relaxes those muscles but can cause swelling. Alternate between the two methods for the best results.

170.   Believe it or not, office workers often have the most back pain. Tight hamstrings are a huge cause of pain in the lower back. When you stand up, your tight hamstrings pull suddenly on your pelvis and lead to lower back pain. Alleviate this pain by stretching your hamstrings.

171.   When trying to find a chiropractor, make sure that you ensure that your insurance company approves chiropractic care. Many insurance companies require a physician referral before they will cover chiropractic care. Additionally, many insurance companies limit the number of visits to a chiropractor each year. Therefore, it is important that you talk with your insurance company.

172.   Call your insurance company before going to your chiropractor. No every insurance plan covers chiropractic care. Make sure you know what your insurance covers prior to being surprised afterwards. Be sure to also ask how many appointments you are allowed to have in any given year. There are often maximums.

173.   When you are lifting items from the floor, you should never bend down with your back and pick them up. Doing this can cause damage to your back, so avoid it at all costs. The best

method for picking up things is to bend your knees, squat and lift it up.

174.    Do your research online to find the best chiropractor around. These days, there's so much that you can learn from a little web research. There are forums and review sites that will give you the low down on different doctors and what to expect. This research can definitely help you make the right call.

175.    When choosing a chiropractor, avoid chiropractors who regularly order or perform x-ray exams of their patients. Most patients who see a chiropractor do not need these x-rays. Be particularly wary of x-ray examinations of the whole spine. The diagnostic value of this practice is doubtful and it also involves a great amount of radiation.

176.    Deep breathing can be a great way to reduce your back pain. Start by taking full, deep breathes. Try holding them as long as possible. Then, exhale them as much as you can. Repeat these exercises at least five times, and try to do them regularly. The best times to do these breathing exercises are after you wake up and before you go to bed.

177.    Birth processes that are used today can cause chiropractic problems in infants. Traumatic birth syndrome results when subluxation of the spine is created during birth. This causes damage to the neck and the nervous system of newborn babies. For this reason, it is very important to have your baby checked by a chiropractor early on.

178.    Babies born with subluxation of the spine suffer a number of problems. Many of these may take a long time to manifest. Some newborns who have suffered birth trauma receive severe brain stem and spinal cord injury. This can result in swelling and bleeding in the brain, trouble breathing and neurological problems. For this reason, chiropractors recommend following a natural birth process and having your baby checked by a chiropractor early on.

179.    Consult a lot of chiropractors before settling on one. While there are many chiropractors who can do adjustments, it's important that you talk to a few before you find the one that's best suited to you. Compare experience levels and your rapport with each chiropractor before settling down on one.

180.    Before having a new chiropractor work on you, it is best to arrange a meeting first to get to

know them. A chiropractor can change your life. The wrong chiropractor can have a very opposite effect. Search for someone whom you can trust. Personally meet with a potential chiropractor before you seek any further treatment from their practice.

181.    Before any chiropractic manipulation is administered, you should have an x-ray or MRI taken in order to rule out fractures, injuries to the arteries, etc. Once you've been properly examined, you'll be able to get the kind of care you need. If this doesn't happen on the first visit, don't let them manipulate your spine. Try making an appointment with a different chiropractor.

182.    When you first wake in the morning, you should allow your back to wake up slowly, especially if you have musculoskeletal problems. Do some gentle stretching and use your arms to support your body as you rise. Then let your legs swing down to the floor.

183.    Ask a chiropractor about alternate treatments if chiropractic care does not seem to be helping. Some pain can be ongoing and downright debilitating. If seeing a chiropractor has not gotten rid of the worst of your pain, ask

about alternatives. Medication or even surgery could be necessary. Explore your options.

184.   Before making an appointment with chiropractor, contact your insurance company and find out whether or not chiropractic care is covered under your plan. By understanding which costs are covered and which are not, you can avoid any unwelcome surprises when it comes time to pay for the services you have received.

185.   When you are reaching for an item that is higher than the level of your shoulders, always use a sturdy step stool or something you can step up on. Reaching up high for heavy or awkward to handle items puts you at risk for hurting your neck or your lower back.

186.   After you've visited a chiropractor, sleep will be your best friend. However, you should be aware of some things first. Never use any sort of pillow that leans your head forward. This puts a strain on your neck. Additionally, do not sleep on the stomach. That can be injurious to the neck and back.

187.   Ask your doctor what type of stretching he or she recommends between visits. Half of

chiropractic care happens on the outside of the office. It's up to you, in your own home, to make the best of your time with the chiropractor. Be sure to stretch and exercise. It'll make a big difference.

188.   Chiropractic care focuses on your skeletal and nervous system and the functioning of your brain. The central nervous system and brain control all the functions of your body, so regular chiropractic care can lead to excellent overall health. When your central nervous system is functioning properly, all of your autonomic functions, such as heartbeat, breathing and digestion work unimpeded.

189.   When choosing a chiropractor, avoid chiropractors who regularly order or perform x-ray exams of their patients. Most patients who see a chiropractor do not need these x-rays. Be particularly wary of x-ray examinations of the whole spine. The diagnostic value of this practice is doubtful and it also involves a great amount of radiation.

190.   To find a reputable chiropractor, ask about treatment methods. Chiropractors who use scientifically based methods use ice packs or heat as well as ultrasound treatments and similar

strategies to those used by physical therapists. Along with an exercise program at home, this treatment should yield significant advancement within just a handful of visits.

191.   Most chiropractors have specialties that they can treat exceptionally well. Find out if your chiropractor has any specialty training. There may be a limit to their effectiveness. Look for a chiropractor that sticks to the basics.

192.   Watch when carrying your purse that you do it properly to avoid pain to your back, neck and shoulders. Work on alternating shoulders often. Don't carry too many things in your purse. It should not be too heavy. Lighten the load any way you can.

193.   Sleeping on your back is the best way to keep your back from feeling pain. To complement chiropractic care, put a pillow beneath the shoulders and head, and roll up a towel to place beneath your neck, and then place a pillow beneath your knees. This keeps your three primary curves supported.

194.   You may be able to save a great deal of money by seeing a chiropractor. Not only are qualified chiropractors more reasonably priced

than medical doctors, their treatments help you avoid ill health. Your chiropractor can provide you with adjustments that will ensure that all your systems are properly aligned and in good working order. This saves you medical costs in the long run.

195.    When you are applying heat to your back, moist heat is best. You can hop into a warm shower and stand beneath the hot water, or you can put a heating pad in a plastic sack. Cover the sack with a damp cloth, and then turn on the heating pad to generate moist heat.

196.    You might be under the false impression that an office worker would experience more back pain in the lower area than someone who is a laborer. The cause could be that your hamstrings are too tight. Being on your feet too much can result in the hamstring pulling on the pelvis. Stretch the hamstrings regularly to prevent back pain.

197.    Ask your chiropractor about the different techniques they use. Chiropractors are often versed in several techniques for alleviating pain. Do some research for yourself and discuss your options with your chiropractor. Ask them for

their opinion on what would be best for you and weigh that opinion against your own.

198.    Every time you stare down at your smartphone or your tablet, you place your neck muscles and bones under a significant amount of stress. Your head weighs as much as 15 pounds, and the more you look down, the more you mash your discs and bones together. The end result is pain.

199.    After visiting a chiropractor it is important to eat a diet filled with vegetables. This is because of the vitamins and minerals found in vegetables. To get the most from your vegetables, eat them raw. Eating a diet rich in vegetables also helps you lose excess body weight which can contribute to back pain.

200.    Add a cervical pillow to your bed. These pillows allow your head to lay even with the shoulders. Standard pillows put your neck in an awkward position because they push your head up. You can also use a pillow beneath your legs to relieve hamstring pressure and strain when sleeping on your back.

201.    It is very easy to injure your back after visiting a chiropractor. This is because a

chiropractor will manipulate your spine. These manipulations will alleviate back pain. Many patients overdo it because they feel so much better. It is essential that you do not lift heavy items after visiting a chiropractor.

202.    Sleep is important, particularly after you have been treated by a chiropractor. However, you should be aware of some things first. Sleeping with a pillow that pushes the chin forward will increase the pressure on the neck, which is bad business. Also, you should not sleep on your front.

203.    To keep your spine and back from experiencing discomfort while you are working on a laptop, keep it off your lap. Instead, place it on a table, at a level where you don't have to lean over and stare down at it. Place it where you can see the screen at eye level without dropping your chin.

204.    Talk with your friends about anyone they've used for chiropractic care. Sometimes it's those close to you that know the best people to call. If you've got friends who swear by a certain doctor, then it may save you a ton of time in searching for the best one around.

205.　Chiropractic care may also improve your immunity. When you have spine misalignment, your nervous system and immune system can be impacted. By having a chiropractor align your spine, you can get more blood flow into your body's nervous system. This increase aids the body in fighting off infection.

206.　When you are lifting items from the floor, you should never bend down with your back and pick them up. Doing this can cause damage to your back, so avoid it at all costs. The best method for picking up things is to bend your knees, squat and lift it up.

207.　Make sure your back is supported when writing on a flat surface. Try supporting your head with one of your hands. You need to take breaks often when writing. You should get up and stretch your body during these breaks. Lastly, make sure the chair you're sitting in is comfortable.

208.　Don't expect a miracle cure. While chiropractic can do a lot, one treatment isn't going to all of a sudden make you pain free. Just like any treatment regimen, it's going to take time, dedication, and patience. Expect to have multiple trips to the chiropractor before you start seeing lasting results.

209.   When choosing a chiropractor, avoid chiropractors who regularly order or perform x-ray exams of their patients. Most patients who see a chiropractor do not need these x-rays. Be particularly wary of x-ray examinations of the whole spine. The diagnostic value of this practice is doubtful and it also involves a great amount of radiation.

210.   Ask your doctor to recommend stretches that would be good for between visits. Being in chiropractic care means you should be doubly serious about maintaining the best overall health possible. Stretching between adjustments can really be a help. You'll start feeling better quicker, and that's definitely why you went to the chiropractor in the first place.

211.   Before you consult a chiropractor, make sure a competent medical practitioner diagnoses your problem. Do not rely on the diagnosis of a chiropractor. Even though there are chiropractors who are know enough to give a proper diagnosis, it is hard for a consumer to determine who that can be. As additional

precaution, ask your chiropractor to talk about your care with your doctor.

212.    To find a reputable chiropractor, ask about treatment methods. Chiropractors who use scientifically based methods use ice packs or heat as well as ultrasound treatments and similar strategies to those used by physical therapists. Along with an exercise program at home, this treatment should yield significant advancement within just a handful of visits.

213.    Make sure that you don't sign any contracts with a chiropractor who orders or performs X-ray exams as a routine strategy with all patients. The majority of patients who visit a chiropractor have no need of X-rays. Full-spine X-rays are particularly hazardous, as they mean significant radiation exposure and have little diagnostic worth.

214.    Before choosing a chiropractor, look into his or her licensing. A quality chiropractor will be licensed. If there is no official license for the doctor you are seeing, look elsewhere immediately. Remember, chiropractic is not something to fool around with. If you wonder about a person's credentials, don't take the chance.

215.    If your chiropractor wants to put you through neck manipulation, ask him for a clear justification. Because neck manipulation puts you at risk of damage to the vertebral artery, it should be a last resort and should only take place when there is a pressing need, so if your chiropractor uses this for all patients, go to another one instead.

216.    If you are suffering from stomach problems, a trip to the chiropractor could help. Misaligned bones in the spine can interfere with the functioning of the nerves leading to the stomach causing it to produce too much acid. So if you are suffering from indigestion or heartburn, consider visiting your chiropractor for assistance.

217.    Consult a lot of chiropractors before settling on one. While there are many chiropractors who can do adjustments, it's important that you talk to a few before you find the one that's best suited to you. Compare experience levels and your rapport with each chiropractor before settling down on one.

218.    When you have back pain and are undergoing chiropractic treatment, make sure you stretch your back before you get out of bed

in the morning. Raise slowly to a seated position, and support your weight with your arms while swinging your legs around to the floor. This can keep your spine from developing further injury.

219.    When dealing with items that are too heavy or large for you to lift, consider pushing them. You can lean your body against the item and push but be sure that it cannot not fall over. You can also sit on the floor and push it with your legs.

220.    If you have a familial medical history of illnesses, a great chiropractor will refer you to a physician to ensure it is safe to perform chiropractic manipulations on you. This is especially important if you or any blood relatives have heart disease, diabetes or lung problems. If you are concerned, talk with your chiropractor before starting any treatment plan.

221.    Call your insurance company before going to your chiropractor. No every insurance plan covers chiropractic care. Make sure you know what your insurance covers prior to being surprised afterwards. Be sure to also ask how many appointments you are allowed to have in any given year. There are often maximums.

222.    Ask your doctor what type of stretching he or she recommends between visits. Half of chiropractic care happens on the outside of the office. It's up to you, in your own home, to make the best of your time with the chiropractor. Be sure to stretch and exercise. It'll make a big difference.

223.    Some people with chiropractic issues think they should avoid all exercises. Not only is this false, but some exercising is actually good for the back; it helps strengthens muscles in the back. So, if you have chiropractic issues and would like to exercise, a good solution is to wear a back brace and listen to your body when it says it has had enough.

224.    Chiropractic care supports nature in helping you attain vibrant health. Your body is capable of self healing when your skeletal structure is properly aligned and your central nervous system is in tip top condition. Your chiropractor knows how to make proper adjustments to stimulate excellent overall healing and health.

225.    Research what chiropractic really is prior to going to a chiropractor. A lot of people have strange ideas about what these doctors do. They think chiropractic does strange things to your

bones or muscles. It's not true. There's a lot of great information online that will help you understand the benefits of chiropractic.

226.    Don't go to one chiropractic appointment with the idea of skipping all the others. Chiropractic is something that you need to follow through on. Most issues take many sessions to work through. You need to be prepared to give of your time. This also means creating a budget for these sessions.

227.    Stay away from chiropractors who market about the warning signs indicating the necessity for chiropractic treatment, who claim to be able to cure diseases, who want you to sign a long-term contract for treatment, market a regular course of preventive treatments, or use fear tactics. Those are just after your money.

228.    Realize that some chiropractic methods bring a high level of risk. Any spinal manipulation that includes sudden movements brings more possibility of injury than other treatments that are more conservative. Neck manipulation can also lead to serious harm and should happen gently to keep rotation from becoming excessive and harming the vertebral artery.

229.    If your chiropractor starts talking to you in big words, ask the doctor to explain it again in an easier fashion. If that leads to more big words, then begin to question the value of the care you are receiving. Shady chiropractors often try to use scare tactics to get you to take more sessions than you need. Using big words is one way they do it.

230.    Did you know you can receive chiropractic care while your pregnant? Many women do not realize how beneficial this can be. The added pregnancy weight can put pressure on your back and neck causing discomfort. Studies have shown that manipulations by a chiropractor can relieve up to 85 percent of back pain associated with pregnancy.

231.    Stay consistent with exercise. One key to a healthy back is flexibility and mobility. Through exercise, you strengthen the muscles around the back and associated with it. By increasing the flexibility of these muscles, you are less likely to put undue strain on your back and keep it from causing pain.

232.    Sleeping on your back is the best way to keep your back from feeling pain. To

complement chiropractic care, put a pillow beneath the shoulders and head, and roll up a towel to place beneath your neck, and then place a pillow beneath your knees. This keeps your three primary curves supported.

233.   Ask a chiropractor about alternate treatments if chiropractic care does not seem to be helping. Some pain can be ongoing and downright debilitating. If seeing a chiropractor has not gotten rid of the worst of your pain, ask about alternatives. Medication or even surgery could be necessary. Explore your options.

234.   Ask your chiropractor about the different techniques they use. Chiropractors are often versed in several techniques for alleviating pain. Do some research for yourself and discuss your options with your chiropractor. Ask them for their opinion on what would be best for you and weigh that opinion against your own.

235.   To maintain a healthy spine while you are asleep, you have to maintain the natural curves of its structure. You can sleep on one side, with a cushion between the knees, or on your back, putting a cushion beneath your knees. In either position, also put a small cushion beneath your head, and position it so it also supports the neck.

236.    Get a chiropractor adjustment if you suffer from high blood pressure. Research study conducted by WebMd has concluded that an adjustment of the neck's first cervical vertebrae has the same effect as taking two medications for blood pressure simultaneously. The "atlas adjustment" in particular has shown great effects in stabilizing and lowering blood pressure.

237.    Add a cervical pillow to your bed. These pillows allow your head to lay even with the shoulders. Standard pillows put your neck in an awkward position because they push your head up. You can also use a pillow beneath your legs to relieve hamstring pressure and strain when sleeping on your back.

238.    It is never too early for chiropractic care. Often children are born with problems such as subluxation. Don't be afraid to have your baby attended by a skilled and qualified chiropractor. Early care while the bones and structure are still malleable can make a tremendous difference in your baby's overall health and well being.

239.    Keep an eye on how you're sleeping on the back to keep back pain at bay. Try placing a pillow underneath your shoulders and head.

Towels that are rolled can help support the curves of the body. Make sure your mattress is comfortable.

240.   If you decide to seek chiropractic treatment, make a wise selection. Just as with all professions, there are good chiropractors and bad chiropractors. There are actually some of them that make issues worse. Carefully research any chiropractor before setting an appointment with him or her.

241.   The way you sleep can contribute to back problems. You should sleep with a cervical pillow beneath your neck. This lets your head drop down, unlike a regular pillow which causes the head to push forward.

242.   Don't be surprised if after a chiropractic adjustment that your body feels worse. It will go away. For some people, treatment gives them an immediate boost of energy, but for others it can seem to worsen the issue. Really give it time. The pain will subside, and you'll start feeling a lot better.

243.   Ask your doctor to recommend stretches that would be good for between visits. Being in chiropractic care means you should be doubly

serious about maintaining the best overall health possible. Stretching between adjustments can really be a help. You'll start feeling better quicker, and that's definitely why you went to the chiropractor in the first place.

244. To find a reputable chiropractor, ask about treatment methods. Chiropractors who use scientifically based methods use ice packs or heat as well as ultrasound treatments and similar strategies to those used by physical therapists. Along with an exercise program at home, this treatment should yield significant advancement within just a handful of visits.

245. Steer clear of chiropractors who want to put you on a regimen of homeopathic products, dietary supplements, or herbal substances for treating disease. If they market these products in their offices, do not trust them. Your best sources for such advice are nutritionists and general practice physicians.

246. If you like to carry a wallet around, don't use your back pockets. Doing that causes lower back strain. It puts constant pressure on the back as well as on nerve connections going to the bladder, colon, reproductive organs and the back

of the legs. To prevent this from happening, just move the wallet to your front pocket.

247.    Never rely on the diagnosis that comes from a chiropractor without independent verification from another doctor. Some chiropractors have enough knowledge to make a correct diagnosis, but you as a patient have no easy way to find out which chiropractors can do this. Talk to your general practitioner to get a diagnosis before going to a chiropractor.

248.    Chiropractic care can help improve lung function in patients suffering from asthma. The nerves in your spinal cord regulate the diaphragm and the lungs. If your spine is misaligned, your lungs may not function properly. When the spine is manipulated into proper alignment, nerve supply can be restored to your lungs. Patients can see up to a 50 percent decrease in the number of asthmatic attacks by visiting a chiropractor.

249.    When you are searching for a new chiropractor, make sure you inquire about the range of conditions they treat. A chiropractor is overstepping his bounds if he tries to treat conditions other than musculoskeletal issues. Try

sticking with those that only treat these ares for someone that's more trustworthy.

250.    Ask your personal doctor for recommendations on the best chiropractor for your issue. Your doctor may know multiple chiropractors, and there may be the perfect one for your condition available. This can save you a lot of time in searching, and it may even get you an appointment quicker than if you cold-called.

251.    To help you minimize discomfort between visits to your chiropractor, apply ice or heat to the painful area. Soreness and tightness are likely to dissipate if you apply a moist heat, through a warm shower or a damp heating pad. To give moisture to a heating pad that is dry, put it in a plastic bag and cover it with a small moist towel.

252.    Before you start getting your spine manipulated, you need to get x-rays done at the office or an MRI so you can rule out that bones are fractured. The cost and minor inconvenience are worth it to be sure that you receive the best possible care without aggravating any hidden injuries. If you see a chiropractor who skips this step, say no to any manipulations. You probably should seek the services of another chiropractor.

253.   Your spine's thoracic area affects your digestion and functions in your stomach. Acid reflux along with other irritable symptoms may occur when your spine's nerves in the thoracic become irritated. When you get chiropractic care, it will help with misalignment problems so that you can have better stomach function.

254.   If you are constantly coming down with a cold, consider consulting a chiropractor. Studies have demonstrated that people who regularly get chiropractic care have fewer colds, with less severe symptoms. If someone has a bone that's misaligned in their spine or "subluxation", it can interfere with the nervous system and weaken their immune system. Chiropractor adjustment corrects this problem and restores proper nerve supply.

255.   Did you know about the potential of chiropractic treatment to help your immune system? When your spine isn't aligned correctly, then this aggravates your nervous system, which in turn, could have a negative affect on your immune system. Having your spine realigned by a chiropractor will increase the blood that flows into the nervous system. This increase in circulation boosts the immune system.

256.   If you have problems with your back, it is never a good idea to sleep while lying on your stomach. Even if this is a comfortable position for you, it can result in damage to the vertebrae. This is because there is no spinal support when lying in that position.

257.   When you are lifting items from the floor, you should never bend down with your back and pick them up. Doing this can cause damage to your back, so avoid it at all costs. The best method for picking up things is to bend your knees, squat and lift it up.

258.   Make sure you protect your back when sleeping. If you like sleeping on your side, keep your neck leveled with your spine by placing a pillow under your neck and head. You can relieve the strain on the lower back by placing a pillow between your knees and bending them. To prevent your body from rolling forward, have a pillow close to your chest.

259.   If you feel tense prior to getting chiropractic care, ask your doctor for some heating pads or warm towels. These should be placed on your back for five to ten minutes prior to treatment. This will loosen up your back, making it much

more amenable to the stretching the doctor will put it through.

260.    Do you suffer from fatigue? Many times fatigue is caused by tense neck and back muscles. By repositioning your back, the nerve flow is increased which allows the muscles in your back and neck to relax allowing you to rest comfortably while you are sleeping; thus, improving your fatigue by getting the necessary rest.

261.    Look for a chiropractor that offers a free consultation. Since you may be having regular sessions with a chiropractor, it is a good idea to know what you are getting into. Use that time to ask any questions and gauge the type of provider they are. If you feel uncomfortable at any time, you should look for someone else.

262.    When choosing a chiropractor, avoid chiropractors who regularly order or perform x-ray exams of their patients. Most patients who see a chiropractor do not need these x-rays. Be particularly wary of x-ray examinations of the whole spine. The diagnostic value of this practice is doubtful and it also involves a great amount of radiation.

263.   Stay away from chiropractors who market about the warning signs indicating the necessity for chiropractic treatment, who claim to be able to cure diseases, who want you to sign a long-term contract for treatment, market a regular course of preventive treatments, or use fear tactics. Those are just after your money.

264.   Remember that chiropractors should not also hawk a bunch of new age remedies. They are likely charlatans if they sell it in their office. Nutritionists and physicians are helpful for this advice.

265.   If you visit a chiropractor who talks about "subluxations," features pamphlets about nerve interference in their waiting rooms, or talks about the ways that chiropractic treatments can help cure almost every medical problem, get out before you sign a contract. Chiropractic treatment is beneficial for musculoskeletal issues, and little else.

266.   Go see your doctor before you set foot in a chiropractic office. Be sure to get a medical diagnosis before visiting a chiropractor. This allows a chiropractor to figure out what kind of methods are going to work for you. A chiropractor might not be your best option. It is

possible that you doctor will suggest some other option.

267.    Before choosing a chiropractor, look into his or her licensing. A quality chiropractor will be licensed. If there is no official license for the doctor you are seeing, look elsewhere immediately. Remember, chiropractic is not something to fool around with. If you wonder about a person's credentials, don't take the chance.

268.    If you have back pain, don't do crunches since they can make the pain worse. You might be better off tying yoga exercises to build core strength.

269.    Ask a chiropractor about alternate treatments if chiropractic care does not seem to be helping. Some pain can be ongoing and downright debilitating. If seeing a chiropractor has not gotten rid of the worst of your pain, ask about alternatives. Medication or even surgery could be necessary. Explore your options.

270.    Believe it or not, office workers often have the most back pain. A cause for back pain is tight hamstrings. Sitting down all day can cause the

hamstrings to tighten. You can avoid this by stretching regularly.

271.    When you sit down, you need to have your knees up higher than the hips. Don't slouch or sit up too straight and rigid. Maintain your spine's natural curve. If you sit in a chair with wheels and that spins, you can do frequent adjustments to your position and diminish strain.

272.    Never take a child to a chiropractor who does not normally treat children. Children are still growing and their skeletons and musculature are quite different from adults. If you think your child needs chiropractic care, seek out a chiropractor who normally treats children and ask them for their professional opinion.

273.    Medical professionals are working with chiropractors more and more these days. Of course, you should always review your insurance to make sure that it includes alternative forms of treatment, such as chiropractors and massages. These services can help boost your physician's care.

274.    Talk with your friends about anyone they've used for chiropractic care. Sometimes it's those close to you that know the best people to call. If

you've got friends who swear by a certain doctor, then it may save you a ton of time in searching for the best one around.

275.    If you feel any sort of pain when you are with the chiropractor, be sure to let the doctor know immediately. Your chiropractor may be an expert, but it's your body. You need to let the doctor know if something that's happening is causing an unexpected amount of pain.

276.    If you are pregnant and experiencing morning sickness, regular chiropractic care can help alleviate the symptoms during pregnancy. Studies have shown that new moms who receive regular chiropractic care experience less morning sickness than those who don't. Not only will chiropractic care make you feel a lot better, but it will also align your spine making your nervous system work more efficiently.

277.    If you have back problems, be sure to sleep in the proper position. A cervical pillow placed under your neck as you sleep can really help. They let the head drop while a regular pillow pushes your head forward.

278.    Tell your chiropractor about any pain you are having, even if the pain may not seem related

to an aching back. The nerves in your back can cause pains in lots of unexpected areas. You may get shooting pains in the soles of your feet. There may be tingling prickles on your legs. All of these can be related to a back issue, and your chiropractor needs to know about them.

279.    Don't be surprised if after a chiropractic adjustment that your body feels worse. It will go away. For some people, treatment gives them an immediate boost of energy, but for others it can seem to worsen the issue. Really give it time. The pain will subside, and you'll start feeling a lot better.

280.    Learn about your back problems from your chiropractor. Generally, what is happening to your spine isn't something that occurred overnight.It's usually caused by damage that has built up over time. One visit will not instantly rectify your issues. Make sure your care is consistent with your care. This also means sticking with your treatment plan. After that plan concludes, go in for regular monthly visits to prevent recurrences or other issues.

281.    Once you decide to take the leap and give chiropractic care a try, you want to do everything possible to verify the credentials of potential

practitioners. Training and professional certifications can be a good indicator of the level of care you will receive. Thus, taking the time to check on these qualifications can help you have a better experience overall.

282.    Don't go to one chiropractic appointment with the idea of skipping all the others. Chiropractic is something that you need to follow through on. Most issues take many sessions to work through. You need to be prepared to give of your time. This also means creating a budget for these sessions.

283.    If your chiropractor offers you herbal supplements as part of the overall care, it may be a sign that your doctor is not on the up and up. Herbal supplements are not something you'd typically see being offered by licensed chiropractors. Do your homework here and look to another chiropractor if you have concerns.

284.    If you are suffering from stomach problems, a trip to the chiropractor could help. Misaligned bones in the spine can interfere with the functioning of the nerves leading to the stomach causing it to produce too much acid. So if you are suffering from indigestion or heartburn, consider visiting your chiropractor for assistance.

285.   Stick to chiropractors that use treatment methods that are consistent with those used by physical therapists. These include manual manipulation but also extend to stretching tight joints and muscles, ice packs, heat and ultrasound. They also feature mixing home exercise with treatment in the office. These treatment plans generally bring improvement quickly.

286.   Watch when carrying your purse that you do it properly to avoid pain to your back, neck and shoulders. As well, don't use the same shoulder for your purse every time. On that same note, avoid carrying a purse that is too heavy or it will cause damage. Lighten your load by taking out things that you do not need frequently.

287.   When going to a new chiropractor, you should meet them before you schedule an appointment. This can make all the difference when you know you're in the right hands. The wrong chiropractor can have a very opposite effect. Trust is key, especially in your chiropractor. Make sure you meet with the chiropractor before you schedule anything.

288.   Be sure to get an MRI and complete x-rays before allowing chiropractic manipulation of your spine and skeletal system. This is part of getting a thorough examination. Chiropractors who do not take these precautions are not to be trusted. Call another chiropractor to make an appointment.

289.   When you experience back pain at home, you can use ice or heat to deal with the discomfort. Both methods have advantages and drawbacks, though. Ice brings swelling down but can make your muscles tighter. Heat relaxes those muscles but can cause swelling. Alternate between the two methods for the best results.